HOW TO DO THE KETOGENIC DIET WITHOUT STOPPING EATING

BURN YOUR BODY FAT IN THREE WEEKS IN A HEALTHY WAY, THE MOST EFFECTIVE DIET TO LOSE WEIGHT

Jessy M. Brown

First Edition

Table of Contents

Introduction: Metabolism

Some people think of metabolism as a type of organ, or a part of the body, that influences digestion.

Actually, metabolism is not a part of the body.

Metabolism is the process of transforming food (e.g., nutrients) into fuel (e.g., energy). The body uses this energy to perform a wide range of essential functions.

In fact, your ability to read this page is driven by your metabolism.

If you didn't have metabolism, you wouldn't be able to move.

In fact, long before you realized you couldn't lift a toe or lift your foot, your internal processes would have stopped, because the basic components of life - circulating blood, transforming oxygen into carbon dioxide, expelling potentially lethal waste through the kidneys, and so on. - it all depends on the metabolism.

Although we think of our metabolism as a single function, it is actually a catch-all term for a myriad of functions that are taking place within the body. Every second of every minute of every day of your life, numerous chemical conversions are occurring through metabolism or metabolic functioning.

In some ways, metabolism has been referred to as a process of harmonization that achieves two critical bodily functions that seem to disagree with each other.

> ### *Anabolism and catabolism*

Our bodies are continually creating more cells to replace dead or dysfunctional cells. For example, if you cut your finger, your body begins the process of creating skin cells to clot the blood and start the healing process instantly. This process of creation is a metabolic response, and it is called anabolism.

On the other hand, there is the exact opposite activity that takes place in other parts of the body. Instead of building cells and tissues, the body is breaking down energy so that the body can function.

For example, as you exercise, your body temperature increases and your heart rate increases. As this happens, your body requires more oxygen, so your breathing increases. If your body could not adapt to this increased oxygen requirement, you would collapse. And all of this requires additional power.

Assuming you're not exaggerating, your body will begin to turn food into energy in a metabolic process called catabolism.

Its metabolism is a constant process that works in two seemingly opposite ways: anabolism uses energy to create cells, and catabolism breaks down cells to create energy.

Metabolism is a harmonizer. It brings together two seemingly opposing functions, and does so in an optimal way that allows the body to create cells as needed, and break them down, again as needed.

Metabolism and weight loss

Let's start with calories: *What are calories?*

Calories are simply units of measure, not real things. They are labels like an inch that really is nothing, but they measure the distance between two dots.

So *what do calories measure?*

Answer: *Energy.*

Your body creates energy from the foods you eat, whether they are healthy or not. Create energy from fruits and vegetables using the same process you use to create energy from chocolate bars and candy.

Although you know that it is best for your body to get energy from fruits and vegetables, your body does not evaluate food. It creates energy from whatever you feed it.

Sounds strange, but the body doesn't care. For the body, energy is energy. You need whatever you can get, and you really don't know that some foods are healthier than others. It's like a garbage disposal: it takes what you put on the ground, whether it falls or not.

So let's apply this to the body and weight gain. When the body receives a calorie it must do something with that energy. If a carrot adds 100 calories to your body, you have to accept those 100 calories. The same goes for the 200 calories of chocolate bars and candy.

The body does one of two things with energy, or metabolizes it through anabolism, or metabolizes it through catabolism. That is, it either converts energy (calories) into cells/tissue, or it uses that energy (calories) to break down cells.

When there is an excess of energy, and the body cannot use it to meet the needs of the moment, it will be forced to create cells with that extra energy. He's got to do it.

You don't necessarily want to, but after realizing that energy can't be used to do anything (like help exercise or digest food), you have to turn it into cells through anabolism.

What about those extra cells? Yeah, you guessed it: added weight.

In short, the whole calorie/metabolism/weight gain issue is really about excess energy. When there are too many calories in the body, they turn into fat.

Sometimes those extra calories turn into muscle. In fact, muscles require calories to maintain their mass, so people with strong muscle tone burn calories without doing anything; their metabolism burns them for them.

This is the main reason why exercise

and lean muscle building is part of a general program to boost your metabolism. The more lean muscle you have, the more places excess calories can go before they turn into fat.

> ### ➤ *Something extra about fat cells*

There's a nasty rumor that fat cells are permanent. Unfortunately, the rumor is true. Most experts agree that once fat cells are created, they are permanent. But this does not mean pessimism for those of us who could bear to lose a few pounds. Although experts believe that fat cells are permanent, they also agree that fat cells can be reduced. So even if the number of fat cells in your body remains the same, your size, appearance, and percentage of your total weight may be reduced.

Tips and techniques

Chances are you've tried to increase your metabolism at least once in your life. Maybe you weren't quite sure what a metabolism was, or didn't know how to achieve your goals.

Maybe you started a rigorous jogging and muscle toning exercise program. Or, he began eating several small portions a day, rather than three large traditional meal-sized portions. Maybe you started taking all kinds of supplements that promised to increase your metabolism.

The thing is, all these methods can work.

Exercise, eating strategically, and making sure your body has adequate supplements for catabolism are three of the many weight-loss ideas that are generally good.

So what's the problem?

The problem is that many of us do not have a real scientific understanding of what, how or why these methods stimulate metabolism.

For example, a person may begin a vigorous exercise program that includes significant cardiovascular aerobic movements, such as jogging or bicycling. After a week, that person may notice a weight loss.

But is this due to an increase in metabolism? Maybe yes, maybe no. Could it be due to water loss through perspiration that hasn't been properly replaced? Maybe yes, maybe no.

Many people risk their health because they don't understand the tips, strategies and techniques to improve their metabolism. The popular and widely respected online publication i-Village highlights 11 key ways to accelerate metabolism. To make them easier to present and discuss here, we have taken these 11 key ideas and divided them into 3 broad categories:

- ✓ Exercise
- ✓ Lifestyle
- ✓ Diet

As you go through each of the 11 key points, you will notice that there is some overlap between them. For example, it's hard to imagine that introducing exercise into your life isn't, a lifestyle choice.

Don't get stuck in the categories; they are only provided to help organize these points, and to help you refer to them easily in the future. The important thing is to understand each of the 14 points, and evaluate how you can integrate them responsibly into your life.

Exercises

Exercise is an important part of stimulating your metabolism and burning calories.

Unless you are born with one of those unusually active metabolisms, which allows you to eat thousands of calories a day without gaining weight, you are like the vast majority of us who need to give our metabolisms a little kick.

Cardiovascular (aerobic) exercise is an important part of stimulating your metabolism. Increased heart rate, blood circulation, body temperature, and oxygen intake or carbon dioxide exchange all send messages to your metabolic system to initiate catabolism (breaking down cells and using them as an energy source).

> ➤ *Build Muscle*

Many people, especially women, are very suspicious about an exercise regimen that can lead to muscle development. There is a perception that muscle building leads to muscle mass, and within a short time, you will look like a bodybuilder.

As long as women aren't supplementing their workouts with specific muscle-building supplements, there's no need to worry, because building lean muscle won't make them bulkier.

But why worry about building muscle in the first place?

Because a pound of muscle burns more calories than a pound of fat. So the more muscle you have, the more calories you burn. You don't even have to do anything. You will simply burn more calories, because muscle requires a greater investment of energy.

But if you build muscle and then leave it without exercising, over time, the muscle fibers weaken and you'll lose that wonderful factory that burns calories.

➢ *Interval training*

The basic principle of weight loss behind exercise is catabolism.

Essentially, if you can design your body to require more energy, your body will fulfill breaking down cells to deliver it. And the metabolism process burns calories.

So, based on that logic, interval training fits into the overall plan. Interval training is simply adding a high energy burning component to your exercise plan infrequently, or at intervals.

For example, if you can jog for 20 minutes every other day, you are boosting your metabolism and burning calories/energy. But you can actually burn disproportionately more calories if, during those 20 minutes of jogging, you add a 30-second or 1-minute sprint.

Why is that? Because during these 30 seconds or 1 minute, you give your body a little jolt.

It's not an unhealthy shake, but enough for your body to have to turn things upside down. And to offset your additional energy needs, your body will burn more calories.

Interval training only works when it is interval training. The benefits you enjoy as a result of interval training are mainly due to the fact that your body suddenly needs to find more energy.

As you progressed and met your energy needs during cardiovascular exercise, you suddenly need to hold on to something else for 30 seconds or a minute; and in that period, it will stimulate your metabolism even more.

If you decided to extend your 30-second or 1-minute sprint to a 20-minute sprint, you simply wouldn't experience all the benefits.

Yes, your body would use more energy

if it extended to the highest range of your aerobic training zone. But your body won't necessarily get that jolt that only comes from interval training.

So remember: your goal with interval training is to give your body a healthy shake where it suddenly says to itself:

"Whoa! We need more energy here fast, this person has increased his heart rate from 180 beats per minute to 190 beats per minute. We go to any available cell, like those fat cells in the waist, and we break them down through catabolism so that this person can get the energy he needs.

Interval training may last longer than 30 seconds or one minute. Some experts suggest that you can use interval training for 30-40 minutes, depending on your health status and the appearance of your overall exercise regimen.

The reason why we focus on a time of 30 seconds to 1 minute is simply so that you clearly understand that interval training is a kind of mini training within a training program.

And, as always, don't overdo your interval training. Your goal here is to be healthier and stronger, and lose weight in that process.

You don't earn anything if you run so fast or ride such a hard bike during training at intervals that you hurt yourself. In fact, it will undermine your own health and you may have to stop exercising while torn muscles or other ailments heal.

Variety of exercises

There are some easy ways to add variety to your exercise program. In addition to interval training, you can divide a longer routine into smaller parts.

For example, instead of committing to a training of 1x1 hour a day, it can be divided into 2x30 minute workouts; or even 3x20 minute workouts.

You can also get extra exercise in your daily routine by doing things like taking the stairs instead of the elevator. Or start the day with a brisk walk instead of a coffee and newspaper. Instead of parking near the entrance to a building, park as far away as possible and walk.

All these tips provide two benefits that stimulate metabolism.

First, you can make exercise more fun.

While it's important to have an exercise routine, it's not a good idea to have a boring exercise routine, because then the chances of stopping are much greater.

Therefore, adding these new elements to your overall exercise commitment simply helps encourage you to stick with the program. And since exercise is an essential part of stimulating your metabolism, any technique or advice that helps you continue exercising over the long term is wise advice.

The second important benefit of variety in your exercise program takes us back to the concept of interval training, discussed above.

When you add variety to your workout, your body cannot enter a groove. Remember, the body is a remarkable work, and you will always strive to do things efficiently.

Naturally, the overall state of your health, which may be influenced by genetics and other factors beyond your control, will play a role in the efficiency of your body.

But no matter how your body is united, you want to do things as efficiently as possible. So when you start exercising, your body develops an expectation of energy production. He doesn't do it to be lazy, he does it because it's efficient. If your body begins to predict that you need a certain amount of energy to complete a 20-minute jog, but then you run for 2 minutes, followed by 5 minutes of walking, 2 minutes of jogging, and 1 minute of running at full speed, your body may require a large amount of energy to help you accomplish this.

As a result, you may find yourself out of breath or tired as your body strives to meet this increased demand. Naturally, catabolism will be involved and your body's metabolism will increase.

But over time, maybe a month or more,

your body will simply become more efficient. It will become stronger, and will be able to supply its energy needs much more efficiently. Your health has improved and your body has to work less to meet your energy needs.

Ironically, this may actually obscure your efforts to stimulate metabolism, because you want your body to begin the process of catabolism, but if your body is working efficiently, it will not dig into your reserves (for example, fat cells) in order to provide you with the energy you need.

So the trick is to keep variety in your workouts. Many people choose cross-training. It targets different muscle groups, but prevents your body from finding a furrow through which it tried to help you slow down your metabolism.

Remember, your body doesn't read books like this. It's not necessary, and he doesn't care. You have no idea that a faster metabolism is "good" or "bad".

Your lifestyle

Balancing work, family, hobbies and other commitments often means that our lifestyle is not so much a choice, but a necessity, but we can do small things that help speed up our metabolism.

Do you know people who carefully choose low-fat, low-calorie meals, are very disciplined when it comes to resisting Chef's special nut cake for dessert, and yet ask for a glass or two of wine with their meal?

These people are undermining their efforts to stimulate their metabolism.

Studies show that drinking alcohol with meals actually encourages overfeeding, which means more calories that need to be burned or transformed into fat.

Many people are simply not aware that

many alcoholic beverages are loaded with calories, almost as much as sugary soft drinks.

A bottle of beer or a cocktail is a few hundred calories. Wine is less, but still adds its amount of calories. The advice here is not to stop drinking alcohol altogether, but to be aware that you are adding to your calorie intake.

> ## ➢ *Rest*

Most of us don't have as much control over the amount of sleep as we should. Work, family, education, household chores and many other tasks can literally keep us from sleeping the amount of time we need.

Experts tell us that getting enough sleep improves metabolism. People who are constantly deprived of sleep usually find that they have less energy to perform their daily and regular activities.

As a result, sleep-deprived people often

reduce their own metabolism. They simply don't have the strength to break down foods efficiently, particularly carbohydrates. This is a very difficult topic, because many people can only find time to exercise by borrowing their rest time.

For example, after a long day of work and dealing with family and domestic commitments, a person may find that the only time they have to exercise is late at night. Then what should he do?

Ultimately, it's a question of balance. Naturally, if you're willing to exercise and your doctor agrees that it's healthy for you, then you won't get into shape by sleeping instead of exercising.

However, if you steal time from your sleep to exercise, you can actually do more harm than good, because the next day, you won't have enough energy to digest what you eat. The answer to this vicious circle is in balance.

You don't have to exercise every night. Or maybe you can integrate a workout into your life during the day, maybe at lunchtime or just after work.

Most gyms are open very early, some are even open 24 hours a day. You can also get some fitness equipment for your home and exercise there.

If you find that you have trouble sleeping, this can also negatively affect the speed of your metabolism, because you won't have enough energy the next day. Insomnia and other sleep disorders are very common problems.

Some non-medical tips to help you fall asleep include:

- Don't eat late at night.
- Try drinking warm milk before going to bed.
- Do not turn on the TV at night
- Try yoga or other stress-relieving practices.

- Try to take a hot bath before going to bed.
- Don't exercise near bedtime, your body may be so energized that you don't want to sleep.

You must learn to relax

We have briefly noted yoga in the Things to Do list above, and that leads us to another key influence of its metabolism, stress.

Experts believe that stress can send unwanted signals to our bodies, signals that lead to slower metabolism. Essentially, when the body is under constant stress, it releases stress hormones that flood the system. These stress hormones actually tell the body to create larger fat cells in the abdomen. The result can be weight gain and slower metabolism.

Some easy stress relievers are:

- ✓ Walk more
- ✓ Listen to relaxing music
- ✓ Meditate
- ✓ Practicing yoga

✓ Eat non-stimulant foods (e.g., no caffeine, no sugar, etc.).
✓ Refocus on self and de-stress

Therefore, there is a relationship between the amount of stress you experience and your ability to break down cells and lose weight.

If you don't want to relax because you don't have time, your stressed life is probably playing a role in your weight gain or in your inability to lose weight.

➢ *Only for women*

Scientists have determined that the 2-week period before menstruation is a time of first-rate fat burning. Australian studies have shown that women were able to burn up to 30% more fat in the two weeks prior to their period.

At this time, the female body's production of estrogen and progesterone is at an all-time high. Because these hormones tell the body to use fat as an energy source, exercise during this time can really be worth it. The body will be inclined to look for fat cells for catabolism.

Don't hate calories

The word calorie has a bad reputation. We are constantly faced with foods that are low in calories or reduced in calories.

The calories coming from the cake are empty calories, which means there is no real nutritional value that your body can extract and take advantage of. But in the bigger picture, it's not wise for your metabolism to become a calorie evader.

If you suddenly decrease the amount of calories you eat, your body won't try to do more with less. It will not necessarily cause catabolism and therefore reduce weight and fat cells. Instead, your body will try to keep you alive by slowing down your metabolism. He'll just believe that something is wrong, maybe you're trapped somewhere without food, and he'll start to get really cheap with energy.

So what's the end result? If your body needs 2000 calories a day to survive, and suddenly gives you only 1000, you won't start burning 1000 calories of cells that you have lying around in your love handles.

Instead, your body will slow your metabolism. You will really try to get as much energy from those 1000 calories as you can, because you don't want to waste anything.

You'll feel more tired because your body is being so greedy with energy, and you'll devote your 1000 calorie ration to essential systems such as blood supply and oxygen.

Metabolically, you will not burn extra calories. In fact, you can gain weight by drastically reducing your calorie intake.

The other side of the coin is that you should consume a daily caloric intake that is proportional to your body size, type and weight loss goals.

Once you determine the amount of calories you need, you can provide them to your body through healthy and efficient calories. For example, if your body needs 1500 calories per day, and a double chocolate cake slice provides 500 of them, you can see that eating just one slice will occupy one-third of your daily calorie needs, and that's not good.

On the other hand, you can see that drinking a tasty soft fruit made with yogurt and nuts can deliver half the calories, but it provides you with essential nutrients, vitamins and other elements that your body needs to do its job in a healthy way.

Eating several times during the day

After the discussion about calories, it is also helpful to keep in mind that eating frequently during the day can be very good for stimulating metabolism. There are a couple of reasons for that.

The first reason is that people who tend to eat all day long make considerably fewer snacks. As a result, they tend to avoid fries or candy bars that they might otherwise eat if they were suddenly hungry.

People who eat all day do not tend to experience severe hunger pains because they have a constant flow of food that enters the body.

The second reason is that, by eating all day, you are constantly keeping your metabolism moving. It's like having a generator running all the time. It'll use more electricity than if you turned it on three times a day.

If you plan to eat more often, you should keep a food diary that records what you eat and drink throughout the day.

You should know the calorie levels of what you eat as well as overall nutritional values.

Just concentrating on calories is half the job. You need to make sure you're eating enough protein, carbohydrates, unsaturated fats, and other vitamins and minerals your body needs to function at optimal levels.

> ### *Eat earlier*

Breakfast is the most important meal of the day to stimulate your metabolism and help you lose weight. Breakfast eaters are much less inclined to eat snacks all morning. Of course, if you are eating more frequently, you can still eat something between breakfast and lunch.

Studies have shown that metabolism slows down during sleep and doesn't normally work again until you eat. Therefore, starting the day with breakfast is like starting metabolism. In fact, you'll burn more calories throughout the day, simply by having breakfast.

Remember, while eating breakfast, control both portions and content. You don't want to eat to the point of being completely full, because you want to eat all day and you won't be able to if it's full.

At the same time, beware of high-fat breakfasts. Studies have shown that high-fat breakfasts, such as those that include bacon and sausages, not only add a lot of calories, but also make you hungry again, very soon. In addition to having ingested a large amount of fat and calories, you will usually be hungry again in a few hours.

Alternatively, breakfasts rich in fiber take longer to digest and, therefore, the body will not be hungry again for some time.

This is something to keep in mind; and it may explain why many people who eat breakfast find themselves painfully hungry at lunchtime. It's not your "hyperactive metabolism" at work, it's the high fat content, which has been quickly digested.

Protein

Studies have shown that having the right amount of protein in your system can actually increase the speed of your metabolism. It requires more energy to break down proteins than many other foods. The longer it takes your body to break down protein, the more calories you'll use.

Different people will require different amounts of protein on a daily basis. Those who exercise and build muscle will normally need more than the average amount.

The USFDA Food Guide suggests about 50 grams of protein per day for a reasonably active adult.

Keep in mind that some protein sources are also sources of fat. Fast food burgers can provide up to 20 grams of protein, but they also provide a large amount of fat, making them almost nutritionally useless. Make sure your protein source comes from lean protein. Typically, the protein in some fish and chickens is lean.

If you're vegetarian, or just looking for lean protein alternatives without meat, low-fat cheese, legumes (lentils) and yogurt are good sources. Simply check food labels to determine if the source of protein is lean or fat.

> ## *Carbohydrates*

When the body digests carbohydrates, it needs peaks of insulin. When insulin is released into the system, it promotes fat storage and some experts believe it also slows the metabolic rate.

The good types of carbohydrates to eat are those that are high in fiber and those that come from fruit and vegetable sources. These carbohydrate sources do not have a high glycemic index score, so they do not cause an increase in insulin levels and therefore do not promote fat storage.

Conclusion

Congratulations. Congratulations. You know more about metabolism and how to increase metabolic rate than most people. You have learned that metabolism is a process and not a real part of the body.

It harmonizes two essential body functions: converting food into cells/tissues and breaking down cells to provide energy. We learned that the first process is known as anabolism, and the second as catabolism.

In fact, it is the latter process that influences our ability to lose weight and prevent it from increasing again.

And beyond the biological fundamentals, we also learned the 3 integrated aspects of accelerating metabolism and losing weight, exercise, lifestyle and diet. And within each of these 3 categories there were a total of 11 important, practical and fairly easy ways to stimulate your metabolism.

Now is the time to act. The next step in stimulating your metabolism is up to you. Good luck, have fun and enjoy a better and thinner life.

Just remember that everything will not happen overnight and that it will take time before you see a change in your life for the better.

Now yes, I wish you the best in your results, and remember, everything is practical; theory without action is of no use to you. It brings everything you learn into real life.

A big hug, your friend, Jessy!

By the way, when you achieve your results little by little, I highly recommend you, if you want to learn much more about methods of losing weight, my book on "HOW TO LOSE 10 BOOKS OF WEIGHT

IN 10 DAYS QUICKLY", is a book that I'm sure will help you a lot on your path to "good health".

Without further ado, you can find it in the Amazon search engine, like: "How to lose 10 pounds of weight in 10 days quickly" or looking for my name, like: "Jessy M. Brown"... Once again I wish you success in your results!